Gut Balance Revolution

A Guide to Heal Your Gut Effectively, Restore Gut Balance and Restore Optimal Gut Health

By

Dermot Farrell

MEDICAL DISCLAIMER

The information in this book is not intended to replace professional medical supervision. The information in this book is highly effective and it will definitely reduce the gut health issues of nearly every person. In some cases a cure may take place; however, there is no guarantee that physical ailments will be completely cured. Prior to reducing or stopping allopathic medications, do consult with a qualified physician.

Free Gifts

Bonus #1 – Grab Free Books!!!!!!!!

As a way of saying thank you for downloading this book I would like to give you two free books, which are available exclusively for my readers. The free book "Juicing for Health – 35 Juicing Recipes for Everyday Health Problems", is packed full of useful healthy juice recipes and Success Hacks - 31 Mind-Set Hacks to Increase Productivity and Career Success, is packed full of helpful mind hacks for developing a more dynamic and enjoyable lifestyle!

Please go to my blog page and sign up here:

healbodymindandspirit.com/sign-up-page

You will receive the two free eBooks, plus weekly updates and even free eBooks!

Bonus#2 - Bonus Video Series

You can check out my YouTube channel, which has lots of health related videos

You can find my channel by typing in **healbodymindandspirit.com** into the YouTube search and under playlists you will find a play list entitled 'Gut Health' which provides a quick overview of the material in this book. Also there is a lot of other general health information there which you can view at your leisure!

Contents

Introduction

Do you suffer with gut health problems?

Do you feel bloated after you eat?

Do you find it impossible to lose weight?

Do you suffer with food allergies?

Do you suffer with constipation/diarrhoea?

Do you suffer with acid reflux?

Do you suffer with a dull stomach ache?

Do you suffer with feelings of nausea?

If you regularly suffer from some of these symptoms, then chances are that you have some gut health issues. How many people suffer with one or other form of gut health issues?...Probably the majority of people in one way or another, or at least some of the time, after all who hasn't ate too much Sunday roast or Christmas dinner?

But when these issues become noticeable, on a regular basis and they start to take over your life to the degree that you have to make many special changes in your lifestyle, in order to accommodate them, well that's when things become intolerable. Sadly western medicine isn't a whole lot of help here. Your average GP will recommend an antacid or possibly some enzymes and some general health advice and that's about that, other than that you're on your own!

However, there is light at the end of the tunnel, you don't have to suffer with unruly gut health issues anymore!

In this book we shall take an overview of gut health issues and then provide a wide range of advice regarding foods, supplements and general health advice, in order to get your life back on track. If you follow the advice therein, you will either find a complete resolution to your gut health issues or at the very least, you will at last have a handle on how to deal more effectively with your gut health problems, with a significant reduction in irksome gut health symptoms!

Chapter One – Why is your Gut in Such a Mess!!!

There is a certain amount of genetics involved in gut health issues, but by and large gut health issues come about as a result of lifestyle and diet.

From a genetic point of view celiac disease (whereby the body cannot absorb gluten from grains) has a strong genetic disposition. However, a lot of people who display gluten intolerance symptoms have developed their condition largely as a result of lifestyle and diet imbalances, rather than hereditary conditions. Recent research has labelled a new variation on this theme called **Non Celiac Gluten Sensitivity** (NCGS).[1] The good news about this research is that it indicates a negative reaction to gluten but without the severity of a celiac condition. What this indicates, is that for individuals who have developed NCGS, chances are that they can largely recover from this condition, whereas genuine full-blown Celiac's usually have to live permanently with a strong gluten intolerance.

Looking back at lifestyle and how it creates most gut problems, I think it is fairly easy to realise that our sedentary lifestyle combined with a poor diet, particularly a diet which is high in processed and denatured foods, results in many health imbalances and gut imbalances are amongst the most common health imbalances.

The reason why gut health issues are so prevalent is because the stomach/gut region is central to digestion in our bodies and digestion determines health. For example, back in the early part of the twentieth century an epidemic disease broke out amongst penitentiaries and asylums in the USA which was labelled "Pellagra". Pellagra resulted in serious health problems and sometimes in death and it turned out that it came about as a result of deficient amino acids in the diets of the inmates. While it gave the appearance of a sort of plague, once a healthy diet was implemented all symptoms rapidly disappeared!

So digestion is vital for health and we largely forget this. When we think about digestive health, we tend to think in term of our stomachs as the sole means of digestion and our intestines as been some sort of waste evacuation system. But in reality our stomachs simply predigest our food. On average food which enters the stomach will exit within about 20 minutes. Food has already been pre-digested to a small degree via the enzymes in our saliva. When it goes into the stomach, the hydrochloric acid in our stomachs will then break down this food further so that we now have a soup like semi liquid called "Chyme". Up till now all that has been happening is predigesting, as in chewing with our teeth and melting the food down in our stomachs, does not provide any nutrients but rather it makes the chyme ready to be absorbed in the small intestines.

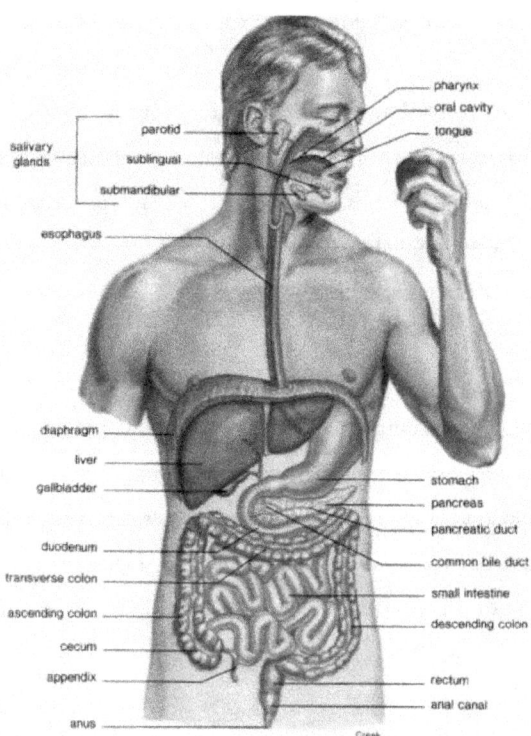

The small intestines are where it's at. In the small intestines, which is misleading as our small intestines are approximately 7 meters or 23 feet in length. It's the intestines which actually absorb the nutrients. Not only are the intestines long but also the intestines containing microvilli, which are small structures which allow for greater absorption of food.

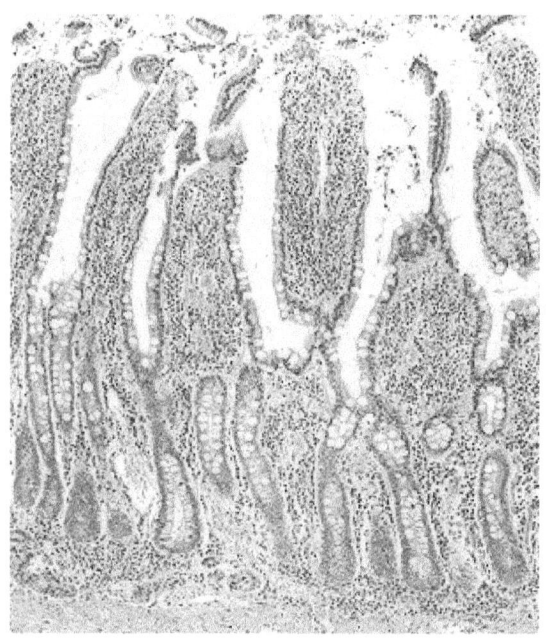

Microvilli – Microscopic structures inside the folds of the small intestines which further enhance the absorbable surface area of the intestines – thus greatly enhancing digestion – many gut imbalances (such as celiac disease for example) impair the microvilli's capacity to absorb nutrients, which in turn results in a wide range of infirmities – remember your only as healthy as your body's ability to absorb nutrients and thus prevent malnutrition from taking place!

So absorbing the nutrients form our food is a complicated and time consuming effort. Some food travels quickly through the intestines, but depending upon genetic makeup and the kinds of food which we are eating, it can take up to several days to fully absorb nutrients from our food.

What is the cause of ill-health in most cases?

Usually the cause of ill-health can be traced back in some way to malnutrition. Now you might be eating enough food, or even more than enough food, but if the food is highly processed and denatured, the net result is malnutrition which can kick of a wide variety of chronic forms of ill health. Once the body struggles to maintain a homeostatic balance, one of the first lines of defence to take a hit is the digestive system, which means either the stomach and/ or the intestines.

One common form of imbalance is food allergies, such as gluten intolerance for example. But also most people have one or more allergic responses to different foods, which are in and of itself an indicator of imbalance. If the stomach is doing its job of predigestion effectively and the small intestines are doing their job of food absorption and elimination of toxins effectively, then most allergic responses will be nullified. Food allergies tend to indicate either a genetic predisposition towards intolerance, to a particular food, or an imbalance in the digestive system.

Some Common Stomach/Gut Health Conditions Causes

There are lots of stomach/gut health conditions which come about as a result of this imbalance.

NCGS (Non Celiac Gluten Sensitivity):

As noted earlier many people who have a gluten problem, have developed it as a consequence of a stomach/gut digestive system which is out of balance.

Acid Reflux:

Allopathic medicine would have you believe that your acid reflux symptoms have come about as a consequence of irregular acid activity, within the stomach, which results in acid moving from the stomach out into the oesophagus, with painful consequences. The allopathic solution is to give the patient an antacid, which settles the stomach by adding in a base to balance out the acid. However, complementary medicine suggests that acid reflux is created by too little acid in the stomach, which results in an imbalance whereby stomach acid comes about in spits and spurts and some of this makes its way to the oesophagus.

Nausea:

Feeling nauseous is very common for pregnant ladies and people who are feel car or sea sick, but some people feel nauseous for no apparent reason, or as a reaction to either smelling or eating certain food. Western medicine has no solution for this other than suggesting an anti-emetic. However from a complementary health perspective, nausea is created by

13

an energetic imbalance in the stomach. In Traditional Chinese Medicine (TCM) there are several energetic meridians in the body, and two of them (the stomach and spleen meridians) directly affect the stomach and can cause nauseous symptoms if unbalanced. Usually the imbalance will come about from poor dietary habits.

Stomach Ache:

There are several causes of stomach ache which includes irritable bowel syndrome (IBS), which is again causes by a stomach imbalance; sudden cramping pains (often caused by constipation whereby food does not digest in the intestines and instead it backs up and creates pressure on the stomach), a dull ache caused by an imbalance of healthy bacteria in the gut, which results in discomfort and a vague sense of stomach upset; bacterial infection which can include stomach ulcers (which are also caused by bacterial infection), which usually results from a lack of health bacteria in the gut. If you suddenly suffer from intense stomach ache, check it out with your doctor as there are some serious health conditions which involve stomach pain, but nine times out of ten stomach aches come about as a result of a stomach/gut imbalance.

Constipation/Diarrhea:

Although appearing as the polar opposites constipation (the inability to defecate) and diarrhoea (too much defecation), are often interlinked and it is not uncommon for individuals to flip around from constipation to diarrhoea and back again.

Constipation usually comes about either because of a poor diet, often a low fibre diet, and/or stomach/gut imbalances, whereby the digestive system becomes incapable of effectively digesting the food.

Diarrheal tends to come about as a result of an unbalanced digestive system whereby the body, in an effort to maintain homeostasis, suddenly evacuates waste products from the gut. We can also see how in some cases the body can flip back and forth between constipation and diarrhoea. Now in some cases, in advanced old age the digestive system is wearing down due to age and this can result in this condition, but other than advanced age the body should not be doing this. So in most cases constipation and diarrhoea are a sign of imbalance.

Leaky Gut Syndrome:

Leaky Gut Syndrome is the new syndrome on the block! It's easy to label our health by saying I have IBS or I have Leaky gut Syndrome etc., but what we must remember is that allopathic medicine likes to label a bunch of symptoms according to a blanket label. According to allopathic medicine, leaky gut syndrome takes place when toxins which should be effective dealt with in the intestines, end up been released back into the bloodstream with a lot of negative health effects. Now while this situation is genuine, what is the cause?

Leaky gut syndrome is again another sign that there is a serious imbalance in your digestive health. Western medicine likes to label symptoms and then promote pharmaceutical treatments, but really most of these conditions can be reversed by simply getting your stomach and gut to rebalance and go back to working effectively and leaky gut syndrome is one such condition.

15

So to summarise while genetics plays a part, by and large most stomach and gut problems are as a direct consequence of lifestyle and diet and can be effectively reversed with some changes in these areas or at least the symptoms can be reduced greatly if not completely reversed. In the next two chapters we will cover foods which should be avoided and lifestyle changes which should be made followed by some great supplements, which will greatly help to restore this stomach/gut balance!

Footnotes

1. J Am Cull Nutr. 2014;33(1):39-54. doi: 10.1080/07315724.2014.869996.

Non-celiac gluten sensitivity: literature review.

Mansueto P[1], Seidita A, D'Alcamo A, Carroccio A.

[1]a Internal Medicine, University Hospital of Palermo , Palermo , ITALY.

Chapter Two – Good Habits for Everyone to Follow

In the next chapter we will get into some strategies for dealing with specific stomach/gut imbalances, but prior to doing so let's take a quick look at the basics of healthy stomach/gut maintenance.

Simple Food Advice

Probably the single biggest factor which causes an unbalanced gut is diet. I think we all know about this but it can be difficult to change our diet. However, at least we have to try and be sensible. Just take a trip down to your local supermarket/minimarket and have a look around at most of the foodstuffs present therein. If you try to take an objective look at what you see, rather than simply reacting out of habit, you will notice that around 80% of the food available is either junk (as in biscuits, cakes, ice creams, sodas and so forth), or it might as well be junk as in its highly processed foods. For example most cereals and breads are highly processed as too are dairy products. Fish is usually okish, so long as it's not salmon (as farmed salmon is often high in toxins) or canned fish.

Meat on the other hand is a veritable war zone of injected hormones and chemicals, so most of this is also junk. So what you are left with is the vegetables and fruits, most of which has been over fertilised and often picked and frozen, shipped half way around the world and stored in freezer for an indeterminate period of time! The average apple available in most American super markets, for example, will be up to six months old!

Fresh orange juice is often made from a pulp, which has a whole bunch of additives mixed in there, and it too has usually been in the deep freeze for a mini-ice age!

And just because it tastes good and appears authentic doesn't mean anything. By and large most foods, even the apparently fresh ones have been processed weeks or even months before we have gotten our hands on them. And even good old organic cannot be trusted. Most organic food is not as organic as you might think. Basically unless you bought it direct from the farm, there is no way to know whether it is really fresh (versus deep frozen for a period of time) or that it really is organic!

I'm not saying this to depress you, after all I also buy food from my local supermarket, and unless you live in a region surrounded by organic farmers, where you can buy produce direct from them or you have big cash reserves, whereby you can buy the highest quality food from a top quality health food store, then you just have to get on with eating a bunch of denatured food!

However, while it is virtually impossible these days to have access to the best quality food, at least we can try and steer things into the right direction. For example, if you have a farmers market near you, try and buy fruits and vegetables there. There is a good chance that the food is not organic but there is a good chance that it's actually fairly fresh. Try and buy organic fruit and vegetables from trusted sources, if you can find them. Also wash both fruit and vegetables thoroughly, so as to get some of the chemicals of off them prior to eating them and finally have a look at your eating habits and try to reduce dependence on processed foods where possible.

While it would be ideal to live on an organic farm and eat everything fresh from Mother Nature, this is probably not going to be the reality for most of us. However, I do believe that even if the food isn't organic and it's probably deep frozen etc., that at least where most of our food intake is home prepared instead of out of a bag or a box, that chances are that it's reasonably healthy. Try where possible to eat as much fruit and vegetables as you can and try to eat raw where possible. As raw food, especially raw vegetables and fruits are high in enzymes (at least some of the time depending upon deep freezing etc.). So at least when we prepare our own food, we are not adding in a bunch of preservatives and additives.

The thing to remember with the modern food industry is that it's all about making money and the way to do this is to make everything appear fresh even if it's not. Think about it this way, if you go into your local store and you buy a fruit or a vegetable that's out of season, then how can it be available unless it has been deep frozen? If you buy a fruit or vegetable, which isn't readily available in your country, then it has been picked from some other country and usually shipped over, in which case it's many weeks or months old!

So one simple way to try and maintain a healthy diet, is to try to eat food according to season, because chances are that if it's in season, then there is a good chance that its actually fresh!

Another thing with the food industry is of course preservatives and additives, so that all those nice tasty foods present in jars, tins, packets and bags are all nice and fresh, many months after they are purchased. So keeping them fresh artificially is good for business, but it's bad for the consumer as we take this crap into our body's, over time toxins build up which make it difficult for our gut to cope with them!

So following on from the old adage that prevention is the best cure, try where possible to eat organic, ideally from the farm and even if this is not possible, try your best to tip the balance over towards eating foods, which are home prepared rather than highly processed, regardless how good they taste.

Finally if we take a look at sources of macronutrients, namely proteins, carbohydrates and fats, we have to take a look at how we are getting these micronutrients. For example in many western countries, huge amounts of bread and dairy products have been the mainstay of diets for centuries. However, most bread today, for example, isn't what it used to be rather it's usually full of cheap starches, even if it appears to be multi-grain, often the multi-grain is more or less a cosmetic after thought. Just make some brown bread at home and compare it to multi-grain, from your local shop, and see how you feel after five or six slices of each and you will notice some discomfort and bloating with the supermarket multi-grain versus homemade. I know that everyone cannot bake their own bread and that supermarket multi-grain, is far better than supermarket white bread, but it's still not great.

Dairy is also questionable, since it's heavily processed versus raw milk and dairy products which have been made on the farm. So I know it can be difficult or even impossible to change these things, but at least we should reduce our dependency upon them. For example, growing up in Ireland, vast quantities of white bread, cheese, processed milk and endless cereals was the name of the game and this is a recipe for gut problems. Because processed bread is starchy, milk and dairy products are full of lactose (unless you are using raw milk which can be hard to get your hands on). So even if you cannot stop taking these foodstuffs, at least reduce your dependency on them.

When I was growing up about 75% of all the food, which I was eating, could be classified under these groups and this sort of highly processed food, combined with a lack of fruit and vegetables in the diet will result in gut problems!

Also in Asian countries rice is very popular which is fine. But rice up to about 60 years ago was heavy organic rice, which was yellow in colour and had a thick outer husk, which is highly nutritious. But modern processed rice has been denatured, in the same way that processed white sugar has been denatured. They have thrown out the outer husk and what you left with as a highly polished, tasty and fairly un-nutritious white grain. It looks pretty but it's not that healthy. So where possible go for organic rice, but most organic rice isn't even really organic. But at least you can reduce your dependency on rice. These days I live in India and a lot of pole in South India eat pounds of rice per day, which is too much. Many of them have distended stomachs, because just like beer drinkers in the west develop stomach distension, so too do many Asian people develop stomach distension.

I'm not suggesting that you give up your favourite foods, but just realise that different cultures have developed a dependence upon certain kinds of food, which has come about historically. But these foods are not the same food which we are using today, so for a start bread, dairy, rice and other cereals where far healthier pre-world war II. Secondly, we tend to eat more foods these days and thirdly we are less active than we sued to be. So because grandpa used to eat a truck load of bread and dairy 60 years ago, when the food was all organic and he worked doing physical labour on the farm for 10 hours a day, whereby his body was like a furnace and burnt off all of the carbohydrates and calories, so of course he was healthy. But now we are eating the same food while leaving a sedentary lifestyle, eating denatured food and lots of it!

Consequently we have to change some of our historical eating patterns, because for a start we don't need such a volume of food. Back in the old days a farmer or manual labourer could easily eat a 1000 grams of carbohydrates a day and burn it off, because they needed 5000 plus calories a day, because of psychical work. If you are a sedentary office worker, then chances are that you will only need somewhere between 2000 to 3000 calories of total food per day, depending upon gender and physical side and general activity levels. So we have to take a look at our food habits and make some changes.

Also because so much of these stable food items are now just junk, probably the easiest way to relieve our digestive systems is to get a little built creative and try to eat a variety of foods, so as to give our gut a chance. If we're eating a pound of bread a day or two pounds of rice a day or a pound of cereals per day or a pound of cheese and other dairy products a day, it's just a bit much for our digestive system to deal with. The simplest way to give your digestive system a break, is to give it a variety of foods, ideally in a balanced way which includes vegetables and fruits. Chances are that when we eat a variety of foods, even if these foods are not organic, that we get a better variety of macro and micronutrients and also it puts less pressure on out guts, as eating vast quantities of the one food, requires a lot of the same sort of enzymes to break it down. So when we eat vast quantities of one kind of food, even if organic, it ends up in a backlog of undigested food in our gut and sometimes even the development of an allergy to that kind of food!

General Good Eating Habits

Before taking a look at supplements for people who are having gut problems, we should first of all remind ourselves to check our eating habits, as it's not just the food you eat but also how you eat which is really important. According to hatha yogis we should chew our food 44 times before swallowing!

I know if we all did this, we would be very slim (because we would not be eating much food) and we would have really big lower faces (thanks to our huge masseter muscles), but on a more practical note, we should at least make a point of chewing our food. I remember when I was young, my brother Tony mastered the art of eating and swallowing a full sized McVities digestive biscuit (it's about 2.5 inches in diameter) in one go and while it was entertaining to watch, this is obviously not a good way to eat our food. Yet most of us do something similar most of the time. In our busy society our tendency is to eat our food in gulp like fashion, as if we haven't seen food for several days and had to satisfy our hanger. Another aspect of modern food eating habits is to sit over our food face down and rat like pigs in a through, we gulp our food down as if are in a race to see who finishes first!

Chew Your Food Thoroughly:

Well these are all really bad food eating habits. While it may not be practical or even enjoyable to chew our food for 44 times, we should at least be cognizant that we are eating our food and chew it according to

23

texture. Something like oats or rice pudding can be swallowed, without any really chewing as they are already semi-solid in nature, but foods like meat, fish, bread, biscuits etc., should be chewed and broken down into a semi solid, prior to leaving our mouth. Looking at Mother Nature, this is what our salivary glands are for. The idea is to have the saliva break the food down in our mouth so that it is semi-solid, then the stomach acid makes it more liquid, so it become a soup like substance, called chyme and finally this liquid substance filters through the intestines delivering nutrients as it goes.

So the first step to good gut health is good digestion, and this means chewing our food. Gobbling down great big chunks of red meat, for instance, is really putting stress on our gut. If we take a look at a typical western styled lunch of baguette filled with chicken, for example, when we gulp this down bits of chicken and bread are sitting in our stomachs and since the stomach empties its content within about 20 minutes, the chunks of bread and chicken are still only semi-solid. No wonder the intestine gets back logged and this can be particular severe on foods such as red meat, which are notorious for festering inside the intestines and take at least 24 hours to digest and sometimes more. This is also why it is good to take a variety of meats, over the course of a week, as red meat in particular is difficult to digest. Also some vegetarian foods are famously difficult to digest with noodles been slow to digest, for example.

Anyhow the first step to gut health is to watch your diet and the second is to chew your food, so as to give your gut a chance to properly digest it.

24

Eating and Activity:

Another aspect of eating food is activity. These days I see lots of people eating while walking, for instance, which makes no sense at all as it makes digestion difficult. Another thing is eating while sitting at our desk feeling stressed. For a start we are probably bent over our desk which makes digestion difficult and worrying or stressing, while eating is a real no no!

From a Traditional Chinese medical (TCM) point of view, we should eat in a relaxed and conscious manner, we should be aware that we are eating and enjoy and feel the nurturing effects, as this boosts both yang (active) and ying (nurturing) energy. While this sounds esoteric, it is in fact a very common sense approach to eating, as conscious awareness helps us to relax, which in turn will relax our digestive system; also we will eat more slowly thus allowing our digestive enzymes and stomach acid to do their work and we will feel more contented, which in turn will make us less likely to eat too much. Often times when we rush through our food, we don't even notice that we are eating and end up eating more. Have you ever ate an ice cream or a chocolate bar, only to find out that the last bite was the tastiest and you wish you had more? Chances are you gobbled down the treat so quickly, that you only consciously noticed that you were eating chocolate or ice cream, when you imbibed your last mouth full!

Water Intake at Mealtime:

Other good food device is to watch our water intake prior to and post food intake. Our stomach is an acid bath and if we drink water either just before or just after food, we end up diluting the acid, which in turn limits the digestibility of the food. You can of course take milk or other

25

beverages, as they will either be acids or bases, but don't take water with your meal as its ph. neutral so it will put the stomach of!

Another good piece of eating advice is to eat less rather than more. In Japan, for example, the people of the Islands of Okinawa are famous for their longevity. There are several factors, which help them live such a long life, but one of the major factors recognised is that they eat until they are still slightly hungry. The brain takes 15 minutes to catch up with the stomach, so if you stop eating when you are full, about 15 minutes later you will feel really bloated! So there is some real wisdom in the Okinawans approach to eating!

Who hasn't eaten too much food at Christmas, thanksgiving or at a birthday party or in a restaurant while on holidays, but let's be honest is it good for health?

Certainly not, as lying on our bed feeling like a beached whale, for a few hours, is not a pleasant way to spend our afternoon or evening and think about the damage which is been done to our gut. The food is simply backing up and been undigested thus making the entire digestive system run badly. You can do it now and again and get away with it, but if you repeatedly abuse your gut, it will bite back with a variety of gut health issues!

Avoid Spicy Food:

Another good piece of advice is to avoid very spicy foods. I know some people love eating spicy food, but spicy food especially if mixed with hard liquor is a recipe for disaster, as it will mess up your stomach! Also another consideration is to balance spicy with non-spicy. In India, for

26

example, spicy food is popular, but so is eating rice mixed with curd (natural yoghurt) at the end of the meal. The thing about natural yoghurt, is that it is a base and it neutralises the acidic effects of spice. So yoghurt or milk are good foods to help wash down a spicy meal, and whatever you do don't drink water when eating spicy food. You Tube is full of entries of people swallowing hot chilli's and then trying to recover by drinking water, well water actually reignites the spice and makes things worse! Next time you eat something too spicy at the restaurant, order a glass or milk or natural yoghurt and forget about the water as it will do more harm than good!

Eat Frequently:

Eating frequently is another good protocol. Although most of us like to binge these days, our bodies actually like to eat little but often. Although this can vary from person to person, as some people do better on fewer meals, for the majority of people eating little but often makes the digestive system run well, it helps to maintain metabolic levels and keep nutrients running around the body.

Don't eat late at night. Back in Ireland it's a popular past time for many people go to the pub and drink alcohol, followed by the inevitable take away as beer encourages appetite. But this is a disastrous decision, as one pint of beer contains around 200 calories, so say 4 pints of beer equals 800 calories, all of which are carbohydrates. Then add in another 1500 calories, in the form of a burger, french fries and a bottle of coke and you are now looking at a days' worth of calories followed by sleep!

This is a crazy idea as the liver goes asleep at around 10pm in the evening. Large intakes of calories, just before sleep, will bloat you while you sleep and leave you hungry when you wake up, for the food hasn't been processed. Then when you wake up, you eat more which encourages weight gain and a backlog of food in the intestines!

The same also goes for non-drinkers. Say you work night shift, well don't come home at 5am and eat a big meal and then sleep, rather eat something small and have a really big meal when you wake up, it will work out far better for your body. The human body is designed to process food during daylight hours, so try as best you can to keep most of you're eating between 6am and 6pm where possible, at a push you can still eat till around 9pm at night, but definitely eating later than that is a serious no no for most people's digestive systems!

Hydrate:

Finally back to water again, do drink enough water, as in at least 1 litter (2 pints) a day, and this could be as high as 10 litters (20 pints) depending upon climate. While some people suggest that water is not important, actually it is.

Have you ever felt thirsty after a meal? Well the reason why is because digestion uses water, if you want to digest your food you have to drink water. The best policy is to sip water throughout the day. Also carbohydrates suck in water. Every gram of carbohydrates brings along 4 grams of water along with it, so if you are eating a lot, you have to take in a lot of water, otherwise the body will become dehydrated!

Chapter Three – Common Gut Health Problems and How to Treat Them

Ok so say you have some gut health issues and you want to improve things, so what should you do about it?

Well first of all follow the advice listed above. Get your diet in order and do all the right things, like eating little but often, chewing your food, varying your food, eating a healthy diet etc. But this is simply the basics, as without this no other strategy or supplement will help, if you are eating the wrong things at the wrong times.

So what else can you do to boost gut health?

Well you can start by taking in some gut health orientated food, such as the following.

Foods Which Are Good for Gut Health

Ginger:

Ginger is a popular food supplement, but also it is a wondrous herb which has many great traits one of which is on digestion. In a clinical study on the effectiveness of ginger on speeding up the breakdown of food in the stomach, they took 24 participants and gave them 1.2grams of ginger one hour prior to eating a meal and then observed how long it took for the food to transit from the stomach into the intestines. Normally it will take approximately 20 minutes for the food to transit, however the average figure which came back in this group was a transit time of only 13 minutes. 1 This indicates that the ginger helped the food predigest approximately 50% faster than normal. What this suggests is that ginger will help food to predigest, which will in turn make for better chyme and thus an easier time on the intestines when it comes to absorbing the food.

Furthermore ginger also helps relieve symptoms of nausea. In another clinical trial on 32 pregnant ladies, who were suffering with morning sickness, they were given 1 gram of ginger per day and by the end of the study 28 out of the 32 women noticed a significant reduction in morning sickness symptoms!2

So ginger not only helps to breakdown the food but also it helps to settle the stomach, in cases of people who are prone to stomach upset!

There are lots of ways to take ginger. After all you can add ginger into your cooking, but one very effective and tasty way to take ginger is as a tea.

Ginger Tea

1. Take 250ml of water (8 ounces) and add in several slices of ginger, taken directly from ginger root. Simply take some ginger root (about 3 grams per cup) and peel of the outer layer of skin from one part of it and then cut of several slices. Take these slices and either crush slightly or blend in a mix for a few seconds before adding into the water. Another approach is to pound them slightly in a pewter, as once the ginger is crushed a little, its helpful compounds will be released.

2. Boil the water and leave to simmer for a good 10 to 15 minutes, in order to get the essence of ginger out. When we think about boiling vegetables versus steaming, steaming is always recommended because boiling takes out the nutrients from the vegetables and puts it into the water, whereas steaming does not do this. However, in this case we want the nutrients within the ginger to come out into the water as we are going to drink it!

3. You will know the tea is ready when a distinct ginger aroma is smelt.

4. Put a tablespoon of honey into a cup

5. Take one small lemon or half a medium sized lemon and squeeze into the same cup

6. Strain the now boiled ginger water into the cup which has honey and lemon present. If you have done a good job, the tea should be strong enough to sting your throat a little but, this means that you really have got the essence of ginger with all of its amazing benefits!

7. Other options include adding in cinnamon and cardamom, which not only add taste but also they add enormous national benefits as well.

Peppermint:

Peppermint has a calming effect on an upset stomach. It relaxes the muscles of the stomach and helps increase the flow of bile. In particular peppermint has a good effect on symptoms of nausea. In a study on the effects of peppermint on post-operative nausea found that peppermint made a significant improvement in nauseas symptoms in patients who took it.3

Furthermore, peppermint helps relieve irritable bowel syndrome (IBS), due to its ability to relax the intestinal walls. Peppermints ability to relax gastrointestinal muscles, means that it is a good way to treat stomach aches, nausea and constipation.

Regarding dosing peppermint is usually taken as a tea and peppermint tea is commonly found in many health food stores and even supermarkets. Of course you can always make your own peppermint tea as follows;

Peppermint Tea

1. Boil water

2. Add in some peppermint leaves

3. Boil for 10 minutes

4. Strain and serve

Wheatgrass:

Wheatgrass is awesome yet underrated herb which can really help gut health. Wheatgrass is simply the grass which becomes wheat, being chopped when the grass is only 6 inches in height. Anyway this grass possesses many amazing benefits which include the following benefits:

- Balances the body's Ph. Levels
- Deoxygenates our bodies
- Protects against cancer
- Boosts red blood cell count
- Cleanses the blood
- Liver detoxification
- Improves digestion
- Extremely high in nutrients including vitamins A, B6, C, K and E, manganese, selenium, copper and zinc
- Very high in dietary fibre
- Thyroid stimulation
- Promotes weight loss
- Strengthens bones
- Regulates blood sugar levels
- Improves blood lipid levels
- Increases athletic performance

Wheatgrass is so potent that it's worth taking as a great health booster and everyone should really take it for a couple of reasons. First of all our diet is very acidic these days, as foods such as cereals, milk and dairy products are all acidic. Most foods which are bases are vegetables, so unless you are eating a truck load of vegetables, your body is probably going to be too acidic. Our bodies are meant to operate slightly into the base range of around 7.35-7.45. The Ph. Scale runs from 0 to 6 which is most acidic to least acidic, with coke and coffee being around 4, on this scale and then we have water which is Ph. Neutral, which is 7 and then we go from 8, which is least base, to 14 which is most base. So our bodies are meant to be slightly base. Our bloodstream has to maintain this narrow range of 7.35 to 7.45, and in order to maintain this level our body will even bleach minerals out of our bones, in an effort to maintain this narrow range in our bloodstream!

Now aside from immanent death, which would happen if our bloodstreams Ph. levels ran outside of this narrow range, even when our body manages to artificially maintain this blood level balance, the body in general is too acidic and in extreme cases this can result in acidosis, where a variety of complaints can arise which includes:

- Fatigue
- Drowsiness
- Shortness of breath
- Headaches
- Confusion
- Tremors

If you have some of these symptoms, then chances are that you either have acidosis or are on the way there. Few people develop full-blown acidosis, but lots of people suffer from borderline acidosis whereby they have aches and pains, feel fatigued and drained and generally their bodies are not working well.

So what has this got to do with gut issues?

Well while gut Ph. level has to be acidic, the body in general should be base, in order to function efficiently. For example, an acidic environment promotes fungal growth, bacterial growth and viral growth, within the

34

body. When we get our Ph. Levels back into the normal range, this bodily environment isn't suitable for funguses, bacteria or viruses. So getting rid of these pathogenic invaders helps amongst other things a healthy gut. The great thing with wheatgrass is that it helps to get the Ph.levels back inline without resorting to eating large quantities of vegetables each day..

Also wheatgrass is high in fructans which promote lactobacilli (healthy gut bacteria – which aid digestion and help to kill of nasty funguses such as Candida, for example) and they also help promote reabsorption of calcium, which promotes bones health, lowers triglyceride levels, which aids heart health and helps to reduce blood glucose levels.

Another great benefit of wheatgrass is its high micronutrient level, which promotes once again digestive health and finally wheatgrass is very high in soluble fibre, to the degree that ingesting wheatgrass can promote bowel movements, especially in people who are having gut health issues.

Wheatgrass is a great herb and will boost your health in general, but certainly it has a great benefit on gut health. Importantly when you initially take wheatgrass, usually it will have as strong effect on bowel movements. So when you start taking wheatgrass at first, don't be surprised if you end up suddenly having to go to the toilet. Fortunately this will right itself within a few days or weeks. The good news however, is that its' your gut righting itself and the reason why there are so many bowel movements is because the wheatgrass is moving stubborn blockages within the intestines. So getting as this 'crap' (literarily) gets thrown out of our bodies, which is really good for health and most people, who have gut health issues, nearly always there will be a backlog, so moving this backlog is the first step towards good gut health. Also for people who are suffering with diarrhoea, wheatgrass will help to balance the healthy gut bacteria which will have the reverse effect of normalising bowel movements!

Regarding how to take wheatgrass, ideally you should grow your own, but this tends to be a big hassle, so while the organic, made at home in your garden wheatgrass is the best, even still the powder form which you get in your local health store, is still pretty good and well worth your while to take it.

To take wheatgrass in powder form, just take two tablespoons (30 grams) of it and add in around 250 ml (8 ounces) of water, stir with a spoon and drink. If you have been having lots of stomach health issues, then take this 3 times a day initially, but when things settle down, take just once a day, as this is enough to greatly promote gut health and health in general!

Apple Cider Vinegar:

Apple Cider Vinegar (ACV) goes hand in hand with wheatgrass in that it is a powerful general health elixir and also it is very good for gut health. The benefits of ACV includes the following:

- Balances the bodies Ph. Levels
- Promotes digestion and stomach health
- Aids blood circulation
- Aids weight loss
- Good for heart health
- Relieves joint pain
- Anti-cancerous

Now out of all these great effects, form the point of view of gut health we are interested in ACV because of its Ph. balancing effects and also because of its effects on balancing stomach health.

There are two factors worth considering here. Firstly, ACV helps to balance the acidic levels within the stomach. Acid reflux is seen as an imbalance in the stomach, whereby acid spurts up from the stomach into the oesophagus thus creating heart burn. However, from a holistic point of view, acid reflux is not caused by erratic acid activity, but rather it is caused by insufficient stomach acid levels. Where ACV helps is that it balances the Ph. environment in the stomach, thus helping to normalise stomach acidic activity. So even though ACV, like wheatgrass acts as a base on the body, however ACV is actually an acid, so while it converts into a base after digestion, prior to digestion it is acidic and it helps the stomach balance its acid levels!

The second advantage is that it works while promoting an acidic environment in the stomach which encourages lactobacilli, which are helpful bacteria which thrive in an acidic environment and help to maintain a healthy gut and help to kill off gut fungi such as Candida!

ACV is very easy to take, simply take one tablespoon of ACV in a glass and add in 250ml (8ounces) of water, stir with a spoon and drink. The only thing to watch out for with ACV is that it is acidic, so make sure you wash your teeth by rinsing your mouth out with some water or another beverage afterwards, so as to wash away the acidic deposits from the teeth. Other than that ACV is easy to take although it is bitter in taste. Also the ideal ACV is slightly smoky in colour because it possesses a string of material known as 'the mother' which is very potent. So when buying ACV try and get the version of ACV which is a little bit misty in colour.

ACV will have a general balancing effect on gut health and is really helpful for people who suffer with acid reflux problems. However, it's not the sort of supplement which you take when you have acute acid reflux symptoms. When you are suffering from acid reflux and you want to treat the symptom take an antacid, natural yoghurt or milk. But get into the habit of taking at least one glass a day of ACV and over a period of a few weeks it will have an impact on stomach acid and gut health in general.

Also ACV goes really well with wheatgrass. I find that washing down a glass of ACV with a glass of wheatgrass is a good way to get my daily quota of both and of course the wheatgrass washes of the acidic ACV deposits form my teeth as wheatgrass is a base.

Kombucha:

Kombucha is a popular health drink, which is basically a sugary black tea, which after fermentation it becomes laden with healthy bacteria, vinegar, b vitamins, probiotics, enzymes and healthy acids (acetic, lactic and gluconic).

Benefits of kombucha includes:

- Gut health
- Weight loss
- Detoxification

38

- Improved immune system
- Reduced joint pain
- Anti-cancerous

In particular, from the point of view of gut health the really great thing about kombucha is its amazing variety of probiotics which help to keep the digestive process working properly.

Kombucha is high in Acetobacter , Gluconacetobacte, Lactobacillus and Zygosaccharomyces probiotics. So kombucha will go along way towards getting your gut to work well. With so many probiotics these will flush out funguses (such as Candida) and aid in digestion.

Also kombucha is high in free antioxidants, which helps to counteract free radicals in the gut, which also aids digestive health. Kombucha has also been known to treat stomach ulcers and helps both to prevent and treat leaky gut syndrome.

Kombucha is a very powerful gut health tonic and one or two glasses a day, will go along way towards improving stomach and gut health. But do note that there are so many probiotics in kombucha that if your gut is out of balance, that initially kombucha might result in symptoms such as bloatedness, gas, mild stomach ache and diarrhoea. Don't' worry about this, as it is the guts way of normalising under the powerful and potent impact of kombucha. So when you start taking kombuhca, ease into it by taking one glass a day for a few days and then build up to two or three glasses a day, then after a few weeks when you feel things settle down, then reduce back to a maintenance level, of one glass a day.

Kefir:

Kefir is a Turkish cultured dairy product, which is very high in probiotics. Kefir has been used as a health food for centuries and amongst its many benefits are:

- Improves immunity levels
- Heals gut problems
- Helps digest lactose
- Kills of Candida fungus
- Treats allergies
- Strengthens bones
- Detoxicant

Kefir's many benefits come from its nutrient rich make-up. Kefir is high in vitamin B12, vitamin K2, calcium, biotin, folate, probiotics and enzymes. In particular enzymes and probiotics make kefir a very potent gut health food.

Enzymes reduce once one reaches 30 years of age, which in turn makes it more difficult to digest food, so eating a supplement which is high in digestive enzymes is a great way of improving digestion. Secondly probiotics are healthy bacteria and healthy bacteria fight of nasty digestive fungus's such as Candida, for example.

Kefir is jam packed with probiotics which includes Bifidobacteria, Acetobacter, Lactobacillus Acidophilus, Lactobacillus Bulgaricus, Lactobacillus Caucasus, Lactobacillus Rhamnosus, Lactobacillus and Leuconostoc.

The result of this is that kefir can heal many gut issues include Leaky Gut Syndrome. Also, interestingly it helps people who suffer from lactose intolerance to actually start absorbing lactose!

For anyone who is suffering from gut health issues kefir is worth trying out. However, kefir being a dairy product, it might be difficult to take for anyone who is lactose intolerant. People who suffer with Candida, for example, are lactose intolerant, so they won't initially be able to absorb kefir. In this case it makes more sense to make an effort to detoxify and clean up the digestive system in the first place. So take other supplements such as wheatgrass, ACV and ginger for a while and then slowly add in the kefir.

Moringa:

Moringa is a tree which grows well in Southeast Asia, and is often referred to as the "miracle tree" because it is very high in nutrients which includes beta carotene, Vitamin C, carotene and protein.   Moringa is so high in nutrients that it has 12 times more vitamin C than an oranges, it has 10 times more vitamin A than carrots and 17 times more calcium than milk, for example!

From the point of view of gut health moringa can help in several ways. For a start moringa is high in antioxidants, which helps to detox the intestines. Secondly, moringa helps to reduce inflammation in the body. Inflammation is the body's way of coping with imbalances in the body; it's a sort of cordon whereby the body cordons off infected areas. For a short time it works well, but after a while chronic health develops. Inflammation in the gut is a real bad thing, as it makes food nutrients absorption difficult and also excretion of wastes difficult. So morninga can help to reduce inflammation through the body, which includes the gut. Also moringa boosts liver functioning, which helps to detoxify the system, which is good as where there is a dysfunctional gut, there will be a buildup of toxins in the body.

Moringa leafs can be used with your meals as in a salad or in a juice, for example. If you cannot get your hands on raw moringa, you can probable get a hold of organic cold – pressed moringa oil. Moringa oil is expensive, but it's potent with about a tablespoonful a day being a really good overall health tonic and of course a gut treatment for gut health problems.

Supplements for Gut Health

So far we have looked at foods which help to cure gut health problems, but there are also some supplements which can help, so let's take a look.

Deglycyrrhizinated licorice (DGL):

Licorice is very good for health and helps cure or improve a wide range of health conditions. However, long-term usage can have a negative impact upon blood pressure levels, oedema and oestrogen levels, thanks to the presence of glycyrrhizin. Whereas deglycyrrhizinated licorice, has all the benefits of licorice but without the potential downsides of glycyrrhizin.

From the point of view of gut health, DGL provides great relief for heartburn, peptic ulcers and gastritis, which relates back to its anti-inflammatory properties and its gut bacteria balancing properties. In a study of 82 patients who took DGL, versus an over the counter peptic ulcer medication, the patients who were given 2 DGL tablets daily, over a period of two years, demonstrated the same level of reoccurrence of peptic ulcers, as the patients who took the peptic ulcer medicine, which suggests that DGL is just as strong as the allopathic medication! 4

They also note noted in this study that the DGL group, just like the pharmaceutical group, suffered from a big increase in the onset of peptic

43

ulcers after they stopped taking DGL. This suggests that while DGL is as effective as pharmaceutical medications at treating peptic ulcers, it only keeps peptic ulcers at bay, as long as it was taken. So for some people who suffer extreme stomach issues, such as peptic ulcers, DGL will probably end up becoming part of a lifelong treatment plan!

Regarding dosage, usually DGL is taken anywhere from 1 to 3 tablets, at a dosage of 380 to 400mg per tablet. Take the DGL tablet about 30 minutes prior to each meal will help relieve your stomach.

With that in mind, it's important to remember that long-term herbal supplement use can have toxic side effects, just like long-term medications can. With DGL, the majority of the glycyrrhizin has been removed, however, a little still remains, so if you decide to use DGL, over a long period of time, do check your blood pressure, from time to time, and watch out for oedema. Also in some cases liver toxicity can occur. Dglycyrrhizinated licorice, is a great supplement and chances are that there will be no side effects, but this is something to bear in mind for anyone who is on long term medication, and DGL been just as effective as a pharmaceutical drug should be respected as potentially damaging to health, in some cases.

As to why you should use DGL rather than using pharmaceutical drugs, DGL being a natural product will have less side effects, but like any powerful herb, some toxic side effects shall still remain present.

And this is something to remember with the various foods, supplements and health tips mentioned in this book. In an ideal world every health condition would be curable, but in reality gut health can vary from individual to individual. For some people, they will get great relief from their symptoms with a few small changes. Anyone who suffers from a strong food allergy can testify to this! However, for some people no matter how many strategies they try, or foods they take, their gut health issues linger on. For people in this group, the thing to remember is that gut health is a complex topic and although a full-blown cure may not come, certainly with patience and application of good healing strategies, foods and supplements, much relief can be achieved.

So if you have tried everything under the sun and yet still suffer with gut health issues don't despair. Things will get better, but some trial and error may be required, and even if a full recovery does not come, certainly a good improvement can be made. The reason for writing this book is to share some resources with you, which you might not have already considered. While modern health care can help in many ways, there is a tendency to treat patients symptomatically by providing different drugs to treat various symptoms. I'm not saying that complementary health care is better, but what I am saying is that it provides us with some more resources and other options and also that it focuses upon balance, where a rebalance can take place often symptoms will take care of themselves!

Betaine Hydrochloric Acid:

Betaine Hydrochoric Acid is an ideal supplement for people who are suffering from insufficient stomach acid levels. As noted earlier from a complementary point of view, acid reflux is as a direct consequence of deficient stomach acid levels, which result in sporadic production of hydrochloric acid in the stomach, some of which ends up in the oesophagus which results in acid reflux symptoms. Apple Cider Vinegar can help to restore this balance as ACV is an acid, but for more severe cases if ACV doesn't appear to help, it's worth trying out Betaine Hydrochloric Acid.

Betaine HCL will help to rebalance the acid levels in the stomach, which will not only cures acid reflux, but also it help to improve the overall health and vitality of the stomach and gut and finally sufficient levels of HCL are required to effectively breakdown and digest vitamin B12, amino acids and proteins!

Regarding dosage a little bit of trial and error is required. Start by taking a meal which contains at least 20 grams of protein (HCL is required to breakdown the protein). Take 1 Betaine HCL pills (around 650mg) and check in with your stomach, after eating, to see if it has made any difference to digestion. You should feel better, but if you feel a burning sensation chances are that too much acid is been taking. If you feel a burning distension feeling, then reduce down to half a pill. If you feel an improvement or don't feel any improvement, just maintain this one pill per meal and after a couple of days try out 2 pills and see how you feel. Keep experimenting with dosage until you feel an improvement in digestion, but don't feel any discomfort. Once you feel discomfort stop and even reduce dosage a little bit, if need be.

So experiment a little bit, until you are taking enough Betaine HCL, to make a good improvement to digestion, without overdoing it as too much HCL will make you feel ill. For most people the dosing of Betaine HCL shall be somewhere between 3000mg to 5500mg per meal. Taking too little won't do anything to help digestion and taking too much will make for an over acidic gut environment.

Contraindications

One thing which you have to be careful about, when using Betaine HCL, and that is when Betaine HCL is mixed with anti-inflammatory drugs such as aspirin, corticosteroids, Indocin, ibuprofen and NSAIDs (non-steroidal anti-inflammatory drug) in general. The reason is that HCL pills, when mixed into a stomach, which is already containing these drugs can aggravate the stomach lining and even result in bleeding of the stomach lining, or even the development of an ulcer!

So while Betaine HCL is a great way to improve acid reflux and indigestion, you have to be careful otherwise you can make things worse!

Also, anti-inflammatory drugs are very popular, ibuprofen for example (Motrin, Advil, Brofen) is a very popular headache pill, and of course aspirin is very popular, so just check out your medications and don't mix these medications with HCL!

L-glutamine:

L-Glutamine is a very useful supplement. L-Glutamine is an amino acid, being the most common amino acid used by the human body (around 30 present of all amino acid nitrogen in the blood is L-Glutamine). Being an amino acid, L-Glutamine will obviously be a big help at building muscle and maintaining lean muscle when dieting, but it also comes with many other benefits which includes:

- L-Glutamine is great for intestinal health, as it helps to rebuild and repair damage to the gut
- It helps to heal ulcers, cure leaky gut syndrome and prevents further damage to the stomach and intestines
- It improves symptoms of Irritable Bowel Syndrome (IBS) and diarrhoea by balancing mucus levels in the stomach lining.5
- Reduces cravings for sweets and alcohol
- Improves the metabolism
- Detoxifies the body (including the intestines)
- Improves blood sugar control
- Anti-cancer agent
- Promotes muscle growth and prevents muscle wasting
- Improves athletic performance and recovery from exercise

So in essence L-Glutamine is a body builder, which in the case of gut issues, it is a body rebuilder, helping to repair gut health issues.

In a study of 20 patients who were fed intravenously for two weeks, they noted that the group, who received L-Glutamine, along with the intravenous food, suffered less gastrointestinal degeneration and demonstrated better permeability than those who didn't. Intravenous feeding has a negative impact upon digestive health, so this study demonstrates the potency of L-Glutamine.6

In another study they noted the healing mechanism of L-Glutamine, whereby it regulates the IgA immune response. IgA is an antibody which fights against bad bacteria and viruses. It also relates to food sensitivities and allergies. So take L-Glutamine will help with food intolerances.7

In yet another study in the Journal of Clinical Immunology they discovered that L-Glutamine regulates the TH2 immune response, which in turn regulates inflammatory cytokines.8 so what this means is that L-Glutamine reduces inflammatory responses, which in turn helps to reduce many gut imbalances.

In summary L-Glutamine can repair damage, reduce food sensitivity and allergic responses and also reduce or even eliminate the inflammatory effect.

L-Glutamine is a must have supplement, for anyone who is facing gut repair issues. Leaky Gut syndrome, for example, isn't just uncomfortable but rather it promotes other degenerative health conditions, such as autoimmune conditions, psoriasis, arthritis and even Hashimotos' disease (a slow thyroid).

49

When we think about healing gut issues, we have to think in terms of getting rid of toxins, righting imbalances and also repairing organic damage and this is where L-Glutamine comes in handy.

L-Glutamine helps with repairing damage caused by a wide variety of gut health issues including Chrohn's disease, Irritable Bowel Syndrome (IBS), Ulcerative colitis, Diverticulosis and Diverticulitis, for example.

How to Take L-Glutamine

L-Glutamine comes in two forms, which are free form, which has to be taken with food for proper absorption. The other type is known as Trans-Alanyl Glutamine or Alanyl –L - Glutamine. This latter time is more absorbable that free form L-GLutmine, so you can take it on an empty stomach, if you want to. You can take it after your meals and in particular it is helpful either before or after workouts in the gym, as it supports both athletic performance and repair of muscle damage.

Regarding dosage, dosage is usually 2 to 5 grams a day, but up to 10 grams a day can be taken. For people with gut health, it makes most sense to take it three times a day, during mealtime either just before or just after food, so as to help with the digestive process. Also for long-term use it is a good idea to supplement some vitamin B12 every day, which helps to regulate L-Glutamine levels in the body, a sot much L-0Glutamine can result in some toxicity, if too much builds up in the body.

50

Side effects of too much L-Glutamine includes increased sweating in feet and hands, back pain, joint pain, muscle pain, dizziness, fatigue, headache, runny nose, dry mouth, gas, vomiting and stomach pain. These are unlikely to happen but it's good to know. The vitamin B12 should minimize the tendency of side effects, but if some of these symptoms arise, then reduces dosage accordingly.

Contraindications: L-Glutamine should be avoided for people who are suffering with liver or kidney dysfunction.

Aloe Vera: Aloe Vera is a super plant which has many great benefits which includes:

- High in anti-inflammatory properties

- Helps relieve constipation

- Promotes regular bowel movements

- Detoxification

- Encourages good gut bacteria

- Helps treat leaky gut syndrome

- Helps relieve heartburn/acid reflux

51

- High in antioxidant and antibacterial properties

- Fights off candida fungus

- Fights off parasitic infections

- Treats mouth ulcers

- Reduces dental plaque

- Improves skin quality

- Prevents wrinkles

So in summary aloe Vera is an amazing plant which demonstrates a wide range of effects. In particular it works wonderfully well on gut health.

Aloe Vera is high in nutrients including calcium, copper, chromium, magnesium, manganese, potassium, sodium, selenium and zinc; It is high in the antioxidant vitamins A, C and E; it is also a great source of vitamin B12, choline and folic acid. Furthermore, aloe Vera contains 8 digestive enzymes (alianase, amylase, alkaline phosphatase, catalase, carboxypeptidase, cellulose, lipase and peroxidase) which help to break down foods. Also, Aloe Vera is high in probiotics (healthy gut bacteria), which help to restore the balance of gut health. In a study on the effect of Aloe Vera on lactobacilli probiotics, they noted a significant increase in levels of L. acidophilus, L. plantarum and L. casei, via aloe vera supplementation.8 Finally Aloe Vera promotes regulation of Ph. Levels throughout the body, which in turn aids gut health.

How to Take Aloe Vera

There is a variety of ways in which you can take aloe Vera. You can take it as a juice or as a capsule. Regarding dosage you can start on a small amount, say 1tsp twice a day taken before meals. Then slowly increase the amount taken up to a maximum of 4 tbsp. twice a day. How much you will take, will vary according to your gut health issues and your reaction to aloe Vera juice or capsules. Aloe Vera promotes bowel movements, so it is a good idea to start of, taken a small amount particularly at first, since it will help to clear any backlog within the intestines, hence too much too soon might result in diarrhoea like symptoms!

Also on the other hand many people avoid aloe Vera, believing it to be a laxative, but actually it is quite safe to take and even kids can take it, but they should take a very small l amount like a tsp. or two per day. Rather aloe Vera is safe but it does rebalance bowel movements and can result in a laxative like effect, if you take too much too soon!

Footnotes

1. Ginger for Nausea and Vomiting in Pregnancy: Randomized, Double-Masked, Placebo-Controlled Trial

   VUTYAVANICH, TERAPORN MD, MSC; KRAISARIN, THEERAJANA

MD; RUANGSRI, RUNG-AROON
BSC.

2. Eur J Gastroenterol Hepatol. 2008 May;20(5):436-40. doi:
10.1097/MEG.0b013e3282f4b224.

**Effects of ginger on gastric emptying and motility in
healthy humans.**

Wu KL[1], Rayner CK, Chuah SK, Changchien CS, Lu SN, Chiu
YC, Chiu KW, Lee CM.

[1]Division of Hepatogastroenterology, Department of Internal
Medicine, College of Medicine, Chang Gung Memorial
Hospital, Kaohsiung Medical Center, Chang Gung University,
Kaohsiung, Taiwan. kengliang_wu@yahoo.com.tw

3. Peppermint oil: a treatment for postoperative nausea
Sylvina Tate MSc BSc (Hons) RGN DipN PGDE RNT*
Article first published online: 28 JUN 2008
DOI: 10.1046/j.1365-2648.1997.t01-15-00999.x

4. Morgan AG, Pacsoo C, McAdam WA (June 1985). "Maintenance
therapy: a two year comparison between Caved-S and cimetidine
treatment in the prevention of symptomatic gastric ulcer
recurrence." Gut 26 (6): 599-602.

5. HIV Clin Trials. 2003 Sep-Oct;4(5):324-9.

**L-glutamine supplementation improves nelfinavir-associated
diarrhea in HIV-infected individuals.**

Huffman FG[1], Walgren ME.

[1]Department of Dietetics and Nutrition, College of Health and Urban Affairs, Florida International University, Miami, Florida 33172, USA. huffmanf@fiu.edu

6. Glutamine and the preservation of gut integrity

R.R.W.J. van der Hulst MD, M.F. von Meyenfeldt MD, N.E.P. Deutz MD, P.B. Soeters MD (Prof), R.J.M. Brummer MD, B.K. von Kreel PhD, J.W. Arends MD (Prof)

Published: 29 May 1993

7. Clin Immunol. 1999 Dec;93(3):294-301.

Effect of glutamine on Th1 and Th2 cytokine responses of human peripheral blood mononuclear cells.

Chang WK[1], Yang KD, Shaio MF.

8. Gut Microbes. 2012 Jan 1; 3(1): 4–14.

doi: 10.4161/gmic.19320

PMCID: PMC3337124

The role of gut microbiota in immune homeostasis and autoimmunity

Hsin-Jung Wu [1,2,*] and Eric Wu

9. Acta Biomed. 2012 Dec;83(3):183-8.

Effect of Aloe vera juice on growth and activities of Lactobacilli in-vitro.

Nagpal R[1], Kaur V, Kumar M, Marotta F.

Chapter Four - Gut Healing Program

Ok so we have covered a lot of ground here in the previous three chapters. We have learnt about good eating habits, which act as a foundation for good gut health; we have learnt about everyday foods with can help to restore gut health balance and we have also found out about some great supplements to treat specific gut health problems. So how best can we use this information?

First of all take a look at chart one and two, as these two charts spell out for you the areas in which each foodstuff or supplement come into play. Just take a look:

Chart One								
Health Foods and their Uses for Treating Gut Health Problems								
Gut Health Basics								
• Chew Your Food Thoroughly • Eating and Activity • Water Intake At Mealtime • Avoid Spicy Food • Eat Frequently • Hydrate								
	Ginger	Peppermint	Wheatgrass	ACV	Kombucha	Kefir	Moringa
Detox			x				x
Rebuild							x
Rebalance	x	x	x		x	x	x
Digestion	x	x		x	x	x	x
Acid Reflux				x			
Nausea	x	x					
Stomach Ache		x					
Diarrhoea							
Constipation		x	x				
Anti - Fungal			x		x	x	
Anti-microbial			x				
Anti-Parasitic			x				

Chart Two				
Health Supplements and their Uses for Treating Gut Health Problems				
	Deglycyrrhizinated Licorice	**Betaine Hydrochloric Acid**	**L-glutamine**	**Aloe Vera**
Detox			x	x
Rebuild	x		x	x
Rebalance	x	x	x	x
Digestion	x	x	x	
Acid Reflux	x	x	x	
Nausea				x
Diarrhoea			x	x
Constipation			x	x
Anti - Fungal				x
Anti-microbial				x
Anti-Parasitic				x

First of all we can see that for any hope of improving our gut health, we must carry out some basics, which are chewing food thoroughly; concentrating while you eat on your eating; avoiding water just before, during and just after eating; avoid spicy food and if you eat spicy food then balance it with a base such as milk or natural yoghurt; eat fairly frequently or at least regularly and stay hydrated. These are the absolute basics. If you think you can take a few herbs and supplements, but abuse your gut by either overeating, underrating, eating the wrong types of foods, or eating erratically at all times of the day and night, then forget about it. Our bodies love regularity, get regular with your eating and eat a balanced diet, is the first step in rebalancing our gut health!

Secondly if we look at chart one, at the various foods which help gut health we can see that these foods (Ginger, Peppermint, Apple Cider Vinegar, Kombucha, Kediri and Moringa) tend to be tonic like in nature. While each one has a slightly different effect, overall the tendency is towards aiding digestion and balancing gut health. Whereas while there are a lot of similarities with the supplements mentioned in chart two (Deglycyrrhizinated licorice, Betaine Hydrochloric Acid, L-glutamine and Aloe Vera) we see that they are more specific in action. Apart from Aloe vera, which is a general tonic, the other supplements are more specific in nature, as in Deglycyrrhizinated licorice, for instance helps stomach acidity, acid reflux and peptic ulcers; Betaine Hydrochoric Acid is great for stomach acidity problems; L-Glutamine is a rebuilder for gut damage.

So putting this altogether we can see that the foods mentioned in chart one should be used as a general tonic, whilst the supplements should be added in to treat more specific problems. For example a person who suffers a lot with acid reflux may take a variety of the helpful foods for stomach problems, but then make a specific point of taking Beltaine Hydrochoric Acid, for low stomach acid levels, deglycyrrhizinated licorice also for balancing stomach acids and L-Glutamine for rebuilding the damaged stomach wall.

The thing is that there is no hard and fast rule as how to take these herbs and supplements. The thing is to try and get a feel for your gut health problem and take herbs and supplements which help with that condition. For example, most people will need to detox there gut, in which case wheatgrass and aloe Vera will be very important. For a person who has stomach acidity problems, for example, they might tend towards taking ginger and peppermint tea and aloe Vera, for example.

So take a look at the herbs and supplements mentioned in this book and use them according to your needs.

The thing to remember with gut health issues is that as noted there are a wide range of possible issues as noted in chapter two. So to rebalance our gut health, we first of all have to make an effort to balance things out and then we have to approach certain symptoms specifically.

Most people will have stomach health issues because they are eating the wrong foods, been physically inactive and also much stressed out. Over time the gut becomes imbalanced. Part of this imbalance is as a consequence of lifestyle and diet and can be readily reversed with lifestyle and diet changes. But more often than not toxins have built up and need to be detoxified. So for most people, the stages of gut rebalancing which have to take place are as follows:

1. Detox
2. Rebalance
3. Rebuild

60

Detox

For most of us when we develop gut health issues we gather up toxins because the purpose of our gut is to take in food, absorb the nutrients and expel the waste products. When our gut starts going out of balance, we stop absorbing nutrients properly and they also stop excreting properly. On top of this, because much food does not absorb properly, even more toxins build up along the gastrointestinal tract. This increase in toxins can eventually find its way into the bloodstream (Leaky Gut Syndrome) and this can result in the development of chronic ill health. Other things which can take place are over sensitivity to certain food groups and an inability to absorb these particular foods.

In a very healthy gut nearly anything can be eaten, whereas in an unhealthy gut most foods can cause some sensitivity issues. Also once toxins buildup, it becomes a breeding ground for fungus's (such as Candida doe example), viruses and bacterial infections, all of which make things go even further out of balance.

Depending upon the individual, this might result in one person having nauseous symptoms and in another person having diarrhea and in a third person having perhaps gluten sensitivity, for example. Often the outward symptom is a consequence of one's genetic predisposition, so the first step for most people is detox, in order to begin the rebalancing process.

Green Tea:

There are various ways to carry out a detox. On one level wheatgrass and Aloe Vera are a really good way to encourage detoxification. Another helpful detox herb is green tea. Green tea is very popular as a healthy tea, but what few people realize is that large quantities of green tea, as in 3 to 5 cups a day, can often greatly help detoxification!

Enema:

Enemas are another process encouraged as a way to detox. In the case of an enema, we place a tube inside the anus and pour in saline solution and then go to the toilet. However, while some people love enemas, from my experience enema's only clean out the lower intestine, because at home using an enema bag it's not possible to get the solution up into the small intestines and it's the small intestines which we have to clean. If we use a large quantity of saline water, the net result is an intolerable buildup of pressure, resulting in a sudden evacuation of the bowels. Although the bowel movement might be big, the result is only a cleansing of the lower bowels.

Another approach is to use a laxative. Epsom salts, for example, have a profound effect on clearing out the bowels; all you have to do is to add in one tablespoon into a glass of water and drink it. But Epsom salts works by filling the intestines with a salt which it cannot deal with and so the body draws a huge amount of water into the intestines in order to clear out the salt. Yes it does produce a big result, but then again it dehydrates the body and Epson desalts should not be taken without drinking a lot of water to assist the evacuation process. Also Epson salts can be really aggressive as can other natural laxatives.

Yet another approach is to use colonic irrigation. With colonic irrigation a machine is used to pump a large amount of saline solution through the bowels with the result of a huge evacuation of waste products or the gastrointestinal tract. However, while colonic irrigation is effective it is costly, embarrassing and useless unless you can do with every other week, because the waste products are only sucked out then they refill within a few days. Colonic irrigation can be used in extreme cases of intestinal blockage, which might be required for some people who are suffering from severe constipation, because they are so blocked up that extreme measure sums tube taken. But this in itself is neither a long-term solution nor should it be used habitually. What we have to do is to cleanse the gastrointestinal tract and then once a deep cleanse has ten place we should maintain its balance naturally without the help of enemas, laxatives and colonic irrigation.

In some case blockages are so serious that laxatives are required, but I personally believe in using natural methods, which are more pleasant and more effective. Wheatgrass, for example, if taken several times a day will often promote defecation, especially in someone who suffers with an unbalanced gut. Aloe Vera is also helpful at getting bowel movements going. One of the most effective ways of cleansing the gut is via water therapy.

Water Therapy:

Water therapy is very simple, all you have to do is take a large quantity of water within a short period of time and it will flush out the intestines. The traditional approach is to take around 3 liters (5 pints) of water within a period of 30 minutes. However, after trying this method out myself, I can say that it is time consuming and uncomfortable as after the first couple of liters or so, water starts backing up from the stomach into the esophagus and one can even feel a little bit noises. Also, drinking huge quantities of water can in some cases end up diluting the blood, which is very dangerous for health!

Anyway, after trying out this method for a week and feeling all of the above I decided to experiment a little and instead of dinking 3 liters over 30 mints I attempted to drink just 1 liter (1.5 pints) in less than a minute, by taking several big gulps of water. To my surprise and delight I discovered that drinking 1 liter of water, within a minute or so, produced the exact same effect as drinking 3 liters of water over half an hour, and without the nausea and discomfort!

By drinking a smaller quantity of water very quickly I managed to flush out my intestines, as if I had taken a lot more water over a longer period of time. Which leads onto the explanation as to why this methodology is so effective? It works by flushing out ingrained and compacted fecal matter from with the intestinal wall. Remember earlier in chapter 1 there are two diagrams which describe the gastrointestinal system. The second of these two pictures depicts the microvilli. The microvilli are tony convoluted structures found within the wall of the intestines. The small intestines are long (around 20 feet) compared with only 5 feet for the large intestine. The reason being that the greater the surface area of the small intestines, the greater the amount of food absorption which will take place. So on top of being 20 feet long the intestines have an even greater surface area thanks to these microvilli. But on the other hand when gut health becomes compromised, the intestines get blocked and even enemas and laxatives can have difficulty in cleaning out the dirt which is trapped in the microvilli.

This is where water is great. If you ask any geologist he will happily explain how powerful water is at shaping the landscape. Water, the softest of physical objects, over time can clear out the most intransient obstacles!

What I like about water therapy is that it's something which you can do several times a week, every day or even a couple of times a day, if needs be. This means that even the most remote parts of the intestines will get cleared out, over time, and furthermore unlike even efficient methods like colonic irrigation, water therapy can be used frequently, without having to embarrass yourself or spend a lot of money. With water you simply drink a liter of water, in a minute or so, and then when the urge comes to o to the toilet.

Atypically several bladder movements will follow, within the next hour and half and a bowel movement will usually come too. If a bowel movement doesn't come, don't worry about it; it will come in its own time. Keep taking the water therapy, do it twice a day, if you need to, and slowly the blockage will become unblocked.

Also on the other side of the coin, if you try out water therapy and find yourself sitting on the toilet for half of the day, then reduce the volume of water accordingly!

Water therapy is a very natural and non-forceful way of clearing out the intestines and maintaining intestinal health. Also as a final note remember not to take water therapy, if you have to out somewhere within the next hour or so, as the nature of water therapy is that it fills the bladder and intestines with water, and bladder and bowel movements can come along at any time, within that hour and a half period or so.

Uddiyana Bandha:

Uddiyana Bandha (flying upward) is a famous hatha yoga detoxification technique, which you have probably seen in action if you have ever either seen a yogi in action or attended a hath yoga class. In hatha yoga there are around 80 main asanas or postures. Uddiyana bandha is a subset of this known as bandha (which means hold) and it is seen as a purification technique, which usually takes place in the morning, but actually it can be practiced at any time. In essence uddiyana Bandha is a detox exercise, whereby you suck your navel in towards your backbone while sucking your diaphragm upward (thus named flying upward). The idea is that by sucking in and up, that the intestines will get a nice massage. Actually it's a really good and simple idea, as our intestines tend to get worked hard but they rarely get rest and never get any sort of massage.

Uddiyana bandha is a sort of the grown up version of rubbing a young child's tummy. Why do young kids like this so much? They like it because the gentle rubbing actually relaxes the intestines. With uddiyana bandha, by sucking in and up the intestines suddenly get flushed with blood which takes away toxins, while putting oxygen and nutrients into the gut. Also it relaxes both either stomach wall and the intestinal wall.

Overall uddiyana bandha has the following benefits:

- Better digestion
- Detox of the gastrointestinal system
- Blood purification
- Adrenal glands become more effective
- Improves liver performance
- Improves performance of the pancreas
- Improves blood circulation
- Increases flow of subtle energy through the body

Uddiyana bandha is a simple and effective way of taking toxins out of the gut, while strengthening the walls of the stomach and intestines, as they tone up in the process.

The traditional way to perform uddiyana bandha, is to stand while holding your hands on your thighs; breathe out and then suck in your stomach and then repeat this process several times. This can make many people feel breathless, so another variation on this is to breathe out and then suck in the abdomen once and then out, then breathe in and then out again. This is a slower way to perform uddiyanaa bandha, but I do see benefits of both approaches.

The traditional approach of doing many repetitions in a short burst of time flushes the intestines with blood, but often it does not have much of an effect on subtle energy. The slower approach works better, both for people who have a less well toned abdomen and also for those who are seeking to move subtle healing energies around the body. As a correctly performed uddiyana bandha will definitely lock both the anus and the epiglottis, which holds energy whiten the body.

To achieve this, when in position try when you breath out, to suck into the stomach and feel the epiglottis closing, at the same time try to suck in the anus. From an energetic point of view, this will do you a lot of good, but it has to be performed slowly.

Another variation is to perform uddiyana bandha on all fours. The advantage with this variation is twofold. Firstly it's far easier for people who are overweight, as it is difficult to pull in a big belly. Secondly, it is far easier to pull in the anus and close the epiglottis, just creating a sort of energetic vacuum or lock, which keeps the subtle energy currents inside the body, thus recharging it from the inside.

Uddiyana bandha is a great exercise, but it tends to be performed in a very flashy manner by many hatha yogis who like to show off their abdominal muscle control, while this looks impressive it does not help us in anyway, as we have to rely on our abdominal muscles and not theirs!

68

That's why I prefer the sitting on all fours method and also taking a more slow approach.

Another even easier variation is to lie on your back and breathe in while expanding your belly. Then breath out and suck in your navel, as if it were intended on making it meet your backbone. This gentle sucking in, will massage the intestines and it's very easy to perform.

The thing to remember about uddiyana bandha, is not to get either excited or put off by watching people in yoga classes or on You Tube, when they perform this exercise, possibly very quickly. The key to making uddiyana bandha work for you is to work at your own pace, concentrate on proper execution and take your time. Also you can increase your amount of reputations over time. Atypically do 10 reps, which is one round, then take a break for a few seconds and then repeat another round and then yet another round. Over time this number can of course increase, but no force should be used.

A Note on Purification:

You might have noticed by now that I am making a big deal about purification and this is simply because when we have gastrointestinal imbalances, toxins build up in the body and the first step in rebalancing everything is to detox the body. Supplements like wheatgrass and Aloe Vera will help, water therapy will help and so too will green tea and uddiyana banda. But one thing which we have to be careful about is detox withdrawal symptoms.

69

Detox symptoms includes:

- Stomach irritation
- Flatulence
- Diarrhea
- Aches and pains
- Lower back ache
- Flu like symptoms
- Headache
- Dizziness
- Vague feeling in the head
- Irritation
- Anxiety
- Anger
- Depression

I know all of this sounds terrible, but the reason for such symptoms is that as the toxins leave the body, they produce side effects on the way out. Don't give up on the detox, but continue onwards as the symptoms will pass away, in a week or two. Also if the effects are too strong then slow down your pace of change. The emphasize here is sustainable change, as there's no point in being a boy scout for a month and then rebounding back into old habits again!

Realistically speaking it's going to take several months to get the gut back into balance anyway, so take it step by step!

Also think about the many benefits of detox which includes:

- Removal of bodily toxins
- Liver cleansing
- Reduction of inflammation
- Weight Loss
- Increased mental clarity
- Enhanced mood
- Improved self confidence
- Improved sense of well-being
- Improved skin
- More youthful appearance

These are just some of the positive effects of detox. But most people fail to make the restoration of gut health, which they deserve, simply because they feel so bad during the detox process that they give up before the toxins clear out. Remember, there is a finite amount of toxins and once they clear out, you will feel a lot better in every area of your life, so stick to it.

Final Thoughts on Gut Health Rebalancing

Wrapping things up then, we begin with detox and then we move onto rebalancing and rebuilding. How best to do this will depend upon your individual needs. Some people need more rebalancing whilst others require more rebuilding. For example, if you have stomach ulcers rebuilding will definitely be required, whereas if you suffer from food sensitivity, then the focus will be more about rebalancing.

The charts above are a good starting point, but ultimately trial and error is the best way forward, once you understand the general principles of detox rebalance and rebuild. You can heal your gut, but to do so effectively will require patience and forbearance on your part.

The good news about gut health, is that unless you have serious physiological damage to the gut, chances are that gut damage can largely be reversed, to the degree that either you will make a complete recovery or at the very least you will have far better gut health than had prior to been obtained!

Finally remember that everyone is different and that the gut is a large part of the body, going from the mouth done through the stomach, intestines and out through the anus. So while the intention behind this book has been to provide a framework which will help you in the process , the only way to really make good progress is to follow the broad outlines, the general fundamental principles, but trial and error and perseverance are required, in order to heal your gut!

Appendix – 28 Day Gut Restoration Program

There are two messages which I wanted to make while writing this book. Firstly I wanted to get the point across that gut health issues can be cured or greatly improved, but it takes detox, rebalancing, and rebuilding. The second message which I wanted to get across is that every person is different and different approaches have to be taken. Even when similar symptoms are displayed the approach required to bring about cure can differ. So the guiding principles (detox, rebalance, rebuild) are universal, whereas the application of these principles is always individual.

With this in mind I have recommended a self-experimental approach and as a rule of thumb I don't like cookie cutter programs. However, I also know that it can be difficult to make a good start of rehabbing our gut imbalances, and a good start goes a long way towards long-term maintenance. While not ideal for everybody, if you want to have a go at making a big splash with, your gut healing program, then try out this protocol. So with this in mind what follows is a 28 day gut restoration program. It's slightly cookie cutter in its approach and there is a certain amount of sacrifice involved also. But the basic idea is to give your body a break from toxic foods and really give it a good chance to rebalance itself. Also before outlining the steps, I suggest that you keep a journal and note down each day how it is going for you and make changes accordingly as everyone is different.

Food preliminaries

Eat	Don't Eat
Vegetables	Most Dairy Products
Fresh and frozen berries	Gluten products
Lentils	Processed sugar
Quinoa	
Grass-fed meats	Alcohol
Organic eggs	Beverages (regular tea, coffee, all caffeine products)
Fermented foods (Kinchi and sauerkraut)	Rice
Nuts	Beans
Seeds	Soy
Sprouts	Corn
Avocado	Potatoes and Yams
Olive Oil/Coconut Oil	Most Fruits

Ok, I know it's very restrictive, but the idea here is to give your gut a break for a few weeks while rebalancing, so try and stick with it as best you can. As we can see pretty much cereals, breads and even potatoes are of the radar. Pretty much this diet is a meat and veg diet, for most people, and for vegetarians it's a veg and more veg diet. For vegetarian feel free to make very big salads with lots of olive oil or balsamic vinegar as a dressing. Don't worry about the calories, in the oils, as you have to get calories from somewhere, otherwise you will waste away!

For meat eaters this is mainly a high protein diet/moderate fat/very low carbohydrate diet. For vegetarians it is a low protein/ high fat/very low

74

carbohydrate diet. So it's a little extreme but do what you can to maintain it for the 28 days. If you start going potty or find yourself becoming very weak and drawn, then add some foods and beverages back into the mix which you find helpful. Naturally there will be a detoxing withdrawal period of around 2 weeks, where you might not feel all that good. Feeling weak, slightly nauseous, frequent bowel movements and headache are very common symptoms. Also bear in mind that the sudden extraction of carbohydrates, from the diet, will also make you feel a lot weaker after a few days, although by the end of the first week you should be feeling alright again. Also for diabetics keep an eye on your blood sugar levels. By the end of this diet your blood sugars may well have improved, but the lack of carbohydrates might make you a little more prone to hypoglycaemia.

Also in particular for vegetarians the diet can be even more daunting. Carbohydrates and proteins result in an insulin spike but fats don't. So changing to a low protein, high fat diet will make blood sugars tend towards the low level which is good, but they could easily go to low. So make sure, if your diabetic, to have a stash of glucose (such as a glucose sweet or drink) handy, especially for the first few days. If you keep on becoming hypoglycaemic, then make a point of drinking some glucose everyday, so as to maintain the balance.

On a more positive note, this 28 diet will very likely result in weight loss and particularly diabetics will see a good amount of weight loss, as the problem with weight loss and diabetics is that they have uneven insulin levels. When we eat carbohydrates and proteins, our insulin goes high and so insulin is a fat storage hormone. When we starve, our insulin goes low and our human growth hormone (HGH) goes high instead, which is a fat burning hormone. So eating a very low carb diet will reduce insulin levels and increase HGH levels. For the diabetics this diet is fairly low protein, more so than the meat eater version, which will increase HGH even more and reduce insulin even more, so fat loss should certainly take place.

Three meals a Day

The detox program is built up around three meals a day. If you wish to reduce or increase meal numbers please do so, as everyone is different and while some people like to eat only one or two meals a day, others feel bad if they eat less than five or six meals a day.

The important thing is it maintain nutritional intake in a regular way. You might like to eat erratically, but your body likes to eat regularly. Also there are too extremes to avoid. One extreme is gluttony, whereby a person eats and eats and eats and overwhelms their system, and the other is whereby a person hardly eats. Hardly eating will weaken your system and over eating will overwhelm your system. As a rule of thumb both approaches should be avoided!

From the point of view of detoxing we are going to approach the three meals as follows:

Detox Meal
Micronutrient Meal
Macronutrient Meal

Detox Meal:

The detox meal is a juice or smoothie and the idea here is to drink the juice or smoothie instead of eating a regular meal. The herbs inside the juice or smoothie, will remove the toxins and also a liquid meal puts very little stress on the gut. Also from the point of view of satiation the detox meal is big, as in about 1 liter or 1.5 pints of juice or smoothie. Also the sheer volume of juice or smoothie means that you're receiving more of a detox!

The Micronutrient Meal:

There are two main meals to the detox and both contain micro and macronutrients, as in macronutrients are the carbohydrates, proteins and fats and the micronutrients are the vitamins and minerals etc. However, the micronutrient meal simply means that this meal is focused more upon providing micro nutrients rather than macronutrients.

The micronutrient meal consists of a large salad, made up of mixed vegetables and with the addition of olive oil and or balsamic vinegar for taste and also for calories. The idea here is to fill your body with micronutrients to help the rebuilding process. For people who feel the need for more protein, some protein can be added, but don't go to town on it, as we are trying to detox the gut! If you eat a big green salad everyday, your intake of fibre will be very high and this should help to move toxins from your bowels.

The Macronutrient Meal:

This is the main meal of the day, where you eat most of your proteins and carbohydrates, it's also the most calorie dense, meal of the day. The idea behind having just one such meal a day, is to provide sufficient calories and macronutrients while also leaving the gut a chance at self-healing, because one meal is liquid and the other is a salad , so only one is a meal of heavy solids!

Finally, I have labelled the meals as detox, micronutrient and macronutrient, but notice that I didn't mention breakfast lunch or dinner. Whereas most cookie cutter programs believe in setting out everything in stone, I don't believe in taking this approach, as some people need a heavy breakfast and very little food at night, whereas another person only eats at night and yet another person has an average breakfast and a big lunch, with no food at night, for example. So rather than me telling you how to eat and in the process forcing you to eat, in a way which is unnatural for you, then this will not do you good.

Rather in this program we are focused upon one third of food intake being liquid, one third salad and one third full- blown meal. If you stick to these three portion per day, it doesn't matter when you eat your juice or your main meal, for example, so long as you do eat them and also you can go for 2, 3 meals or even 5 or 6 meals a day, so long as it is split accordingly. For example, a person who only wants to eat 2 meals a day could skip the juice/smoothie meal and go for a main meal and a very big salad as the other meal, for instance. While a person who like to eat say 6 times a day could go for 3 juice/smoothie meals and then a salad meal, a homemade meal and a main meal for the final one.

I'm leaving all these options open for everyone is different. A person who is 4 foot tall and weighs 80lbs, is probably going to eat less than someone who is 6 foot five and who weights 300lbs, so how can they be treated the same!

Also one person weighing 180 pounds only needs 2500 calories a day, whereas another person, who weighs in at 180 needs 5000 calories a day!

So just remember everything in this gut restoration program is a guide and is not set in stone. Try and avoid the wrong foods, try and split your food intake into one third liquid, one third salad and one third heavy solid and keep it up for a few weeks and good results shall come!

Detox Shakes and Juices

What follows are 3 shakes and 3 juices. Make a point of taking one each day over the 28 day gut restoration period

Juices

Apples/Oranges & Carrots

Ingredients:

- 2 medium apples
- 2 oranges
- 14 medium sized carrots

Procedure:

1. Peel and chop the fruit and vegetables.
2. Mix all together in a blender.
3. Add 500 ml of water and blend for 1 to 1.5 minutes.
4. Filter using a filter and a large spoon so as to squeeze out the juice.
5. Then take the juice and drink or place in the refrigerator for later.

Benefits:

- Apples are high in insoluble fibre. Because fibre can't be absorbed by the body it has to be excreted and it will help the digestion process while doing this. Also it has pectin, an enzyme which helps to break down food.
- The acids in orange juice help the digestion process.
- Carrots help to cleanse the liver and also stimulate bile production, which is good for digestion. Carrots also boost energy levels and enhance the taste.

Basil, Carrots, lemon & Peaches

Ingredients:

- 3 basil leaves
- 14 carrots
- 1 lemon
- 5 medium sized peaches

Procedure:

1. Peel and chop the fruit and vegetables.
2. Mix all together in a blender.
3. Add 500 ml of water and blend for 1 to 1.5 minutes.
4. Filter using a filter and a large spoon so as to squeeze out the juice.
5. Then take the juice and drink or place in the refrigerator for later.

Benefits:

- Basil helps to improve the digestion process.
- Carrots help to cleanse the liver and also stimulate bile production, which is good for digestion. Carrots also boost energy levels and enhance the taste.
- Lemon juice boosts the digestive process.
- Peaches boost the digestive process, and they also taste really good!

Apples, Lime & Strawberries

Ingredients:

- 2 apples
- One half of a lime
- 3 cups of strawberries

Procedure:

1. Peel and chop the fruit. Mix all together in a blender.
2. Add 500 ml of water and add sugar if you want a sweeter taste.
3. Blend for 1 to 1.5 minutes.
4. Filter using a filter and a large spoon so as to squeeze out the juice.
5. Then take the juice and drink or place in the refrigerator for later.

Benefits:

- Apples are high in insoluble fibre. Because fibre can't be absorbed by the body it has to be excreted and it will help the digestion process while doing this. Also it has pectin, an enzyme which helps to break down food.
- Limes boost digestion.
- Strawberries reduce inflammation of the stomach lining thus relieving gastritis.

Smoothies

Banana Relief

Ingredients:

- 3 bananas
- 2 avocados
- 1 cup of aloe Vera gel or liquid
- 2tbsp's of honey
- 1 cup of ice cubes and 300ml of cold water or 500ml of cold milk or 500ml of natural yoghurt

Procedure:

1. Place the fruit and aloe Vera oil into a blender.
2. Blend until smooth.
3. Add some extra natural yoghurt in if you want to make it more liquid.
4. Add sugar or honey if you want to make sweeter.

Benefits:

Bananas: Contain pectin, which helps with bowel movements. Often stomach aches result from blocked intestines which results in the intestines becoming bigger, which then presses (painfully) against the stomach.

Avocados: Reduce inflammation in the stomach lining.

Aloe Vera: Improves digestive functioning thus relieving stomach ache.

Honey: Reduces inflammation of the oesophagus and stomach lining and also it has a soothing effect which helps both with stomach ache and with acid reflux.

Papaya Yoghurt Twist

Ingredients:

- 1 papaya
- 1 knob of ginger
- 3 tbsp. of honey
- 1 cup of ice cubes and 300ml of cold water or 500ml of cold milk or 500ml of natural yoghurt

Procedure:

1. Place the fruit, yoghurt, ginger and cold water/milk/natural yoghurt into a blender.
2. Blend until smooth.
3. Add some extra natural yoghurt in if you want to make it more liquid.
4. Add sugar or honey if you want to make sweeter.

Benefits:

Papaya: Helps to settle the stomach

Ginger: Improves the digestive system and also helps out with nausea.

Natural Yoghurt: Is a great probiotic and helps to fill the stomach with friendly bacteria, which aid in digestion. Natural yoghurt is also a base and helps to reduce acidity in the stomach.

Honey: Reduces inflammation of the oesophagus and stomach lining and also it has a soothing effect which helps both with stomach ache and with acid reflux.

Strawberries/Peaches and Natural Yoghurt

Ingredients:

- 3 cups of strawberries
- 5 medium sized peaches
- 1000ml of natural yoghurt

Procedure:

1. Place the fruit and natural yoghurt into a blender.
2. Blend until smooth.
3. Add some extra natural yoghurt or milk in if you want to make it more liquid.
4. Add sugar or honey if you want to make sweeter.

Benefits:

Strawberries: Reduce inflammation of the stomach lining thus relieving gastritis,

Peaches: Boost the digestive process, and they also taste really good!

85

Honey: Reduces inflammation of the oesophagus and stomach lining and also it has a soothing effect which helps both with stomach ache and with acid reflux.

Micronutrient Meal

The idea behind the macronutrient meal, is to have a meal which is high in vitamins and minerals. With that in mind the micronutrient meal is a big salad. The salads mentioned below are purely vegetarian, but you can add in meat or fish if you like, but do try to keep to light meats or fishes, such as simple chicken breast, turkey breast, salmon or tuna for example. Remember we are trying to ease the burden on our gut, so if you add meat or fish, just add enough to add in some protein and taste, but don't go overboard!

Basic Healthy Salad

Ingredients:

- A handful of kale
- One medium red cabbage/ or one medium sized head of lettuce
- 6 carrots
- 2 medium sized beetroot
- 2 large red peppers
- 2 large yellow peppers
- ½ cup of raw sunflower seeds
- ½ cup of fennel
- ½ cup of sprouted mung beans
- 4 medium sized tomatoes

Dressing:

- ¼ cup of balsamic vinegar
- 2 tablespoons of olive oil

- 1 tsp. of chopped raw garlic
- 1 tsp. of Dijon mustard
- Medium lemon juiced
- ¼ tsp. of salt
- 14/tsp. of pepper

Directions:

The mung beans require a little bit of preparation. Other than that simply chop everything in small pieces, and then add in the various dressings at the end,

Regarding mung beans, to sprout them do as follows:

1). Wash the beans thoroughly in water
2). Leave the beans in a container overnight, with about an inch of water over them and a cover over the box.
3). Next day strain out the water, rinse and refill the water again, and once more leave overnight.
4). Repeat this process until sprouts have formed out of the mung beans, which should take two or three days. These sprouted moon beans are now very nutritious and tasty too.

Kale and Humus Salad

Ingredients:

- 1 head of kale
- 100grams/4 ounces of mushrooms
- 1 large yellow pepper
- 1 large green pepper
- 2 large onions
- 3 medium sized tomatoes
- ½ cup of walnuts or other nuts which you like

Dressing:

- ½ cup of humus
- 2 cloves of garlic
- 1 tablespoon of parsley
- 1 large lemon juiced or two medium lemons juiced
- 3 tablespoons of olive oil
- Salt and pepper to taste

Directions:

Simply slice the vegetables and fry the mushrooms. Then mix in the mushrooms with the vegetables and then add the dressings to taste, mixing everything as you go.

Quinoa Salad

Ingredients:

- 4 cups of cooked quinoa
- ½ a cup of scallions sliced
- 2 large apples (either of green or red variety)
- 1 cup of cranberries
- ½ a cup of nuts of your choice

Dressing:

- 3 tablespoons of honey
- 2 tablespoons of fresh mint
- 1 medium sized lemon juiced
- ½ a cup of olive oil
- Salt and pepper to taste

Directions:

Quinoa Preparation

1. Rinse the quinoa in water so as to clean of any deposits
2. To cook the quinoa, take one and a half cups of quinoa and add in 3 cups of water and heat.
3. After it boils leave it to simmer for 15 minutes while stirring occasionally.

Other than the quinoa simply slice the vegetables and then mix in the quinoa, adding in the dressing at the end.

Citrus and Seed Salad

Ingredients:

- 1 large head of lettuce
- 1 large grapefruit, 1 large orange and 1 medium sized lemon
- 1 tablespoon of sunflower seeds
- 1 tablespoon of pumpkin seeds
- 1 tablespoon of fennel
- ½ cup of olives
- ½ cup of olive oil
- Salt and pepper to taste

Directions:

Simple slice the citrus fruit and add in the seeds and olive oil and salt and mix up and serve.

Mixed Fruit and Berries Salad

Ingredients:

- 1 cup of kale
- 1 large green pepper and 1 large yellow or red pepper
- 1 cup of cherry tomatoes

- 1 orange
- 1 cup of sliced peaches
- 1 large pear
- 1 medium sized bowl of either green or red grapes (ideally red grapes)
- 1 cup of blueberries
- 1 cup of blackberries
- 1 cup of strawberries

Dressing

- 3 tablespoons of honey
- ½ cup of olive oil
- Salt and pepper to taste

Directions:

Just slice mix and serve!

Mixed Veg Salad

Ingredients:

- A handful of broccoli
- The seeds of one large pomegranate
- ½ a cup of fennel
- 2 avocados
- ½ a cup of nuts of your choice
- 1 large orange

- 1 medium sized lemon squeezed
- ½ a cup of olive oil
- Salt and pepper to taste

Directions:

Steam or boil the broccoli until slightly cooked. Chop and mix the vegetables and fruit. Add everything in together and squeeze in lemon juice and add in olive oil, salt and pepper to taste

Macronutrient Meal

The macronutrient meal is very straightforward, simply take one good source of protein such as grass fed beef or fish, for meat eaters, or lentil, quinoa or sprouts for vegetarians and then add in some vegetables as a side order.

The two main things with the macronutrient meal, is to firstly eat enough proteins and fats (we're not too worried about carbohydrates as healthy fats can substitute for starchy carbs) and secondly to satiate ourselves.

The difficult thing with the macronutrient meal is avoiding starchy carbs, which means that unless you eat lots of vegetables, that it can be a little bit unfilling. So to fill out this meal, either eats lots of vegetables and some gut friendly fruits, such s bananas and apples and avocadoes, or simply eat a larger main portion. So maybe two chicken breasts, for example, or if vegetarian cook 3 cups of quinoa and have a really big but simple meal.

Another nice way to fill out the main meal is to either begin with a soup or to make up a casserole or stew, as the mixture of liquids and solids is more satisfying. Below are two examples of dishes which are filling, while also being good for gut health and free of starchy carbohydrates.

Chicken Casserole

Ingredients:

- Four chicken breast with bones (good for health and tasty)
- Chicken stock cubes
- 4 chopped onions
- A small bowl of mushrooms
- 1 cup of sour cream

Directions:

1. Take two chicken stock cubes and melt into a small saucepan of water.
2. Cook the chicken either via frying, grilling or steaming.
3. Take the chicken and the chicken stock and add in the other vegetables into a baking container and place into a preheated oven. Leave in the oven at 350

degrees Fahrenheit (175 Celsius) and leave for half an hour.

Vegetarian Stew

Ingredients:

- 2 onions peeled
- 2 parsnips
- 4 pieces of celery
- 1 pint of vegetable stock
- 6 tomatoes sliced
- Some chopped parsley
- 1 tablespoon of olive oil

Directions:

1. Heat the olive oil in a large pan along with the onions (onions take longest time to cook)
2. Add in the other vegetables
3. Once they are lightly cooked add in the vegetable stock and leave to simmer for a few minutes
4. Once cooked sprinkle with chopped parsley

Supplementation

For supplementation you can add in wheatgrass and aloe Vera for detoxification. Take aloe Vera with every meal and for the duration of the 28 day program take three glasses of wheatgrass a day. Also try out some water therapy, as this will also help to clear out the toxins from the bowels. As always see how it goes and if you find yourself having endless bowel movements, then reduce the intake of wheatgrass and Aloe Vera accordingly.

Another really useful supplement is L-Glutamine, as it's a great rebuilder as well as been a general tonic.

Other supplements such as Kambucha or ACV, for example, would also be a good idea, but the minimum should be wheatgrass, Aloe Vera and L-Glutamine. Other than this, as always green tea is a great detox option which you might consider adding in.

Summing up the 28 Day Gut Restoration Program

As noted at the beginning of this Appendix I'm not a big fan of cookie cutter programs and this is because everyone is different. For example, some people are full-blown meat eaters, others are vegetarians; some pope have serious food allergies and others have no allergies but they have stomach aches and nausea or possible IBS, for example. So there's no way of creating a perfect program.

Also everyone has different lifestyles, with some people liking to eat many meals whereas others want to eat very infrequently, for example. So we have to ask ourselves, when we are considering a 28 detox program, as to what we want to achieve and how we want to go about achieving it.

This is why it has been created to be very flexible, the idea being to avoid foods which are high in toxins, allergic responses or simply hard to digest, while eating other foods, which aid digestion. The daily juice or smoothie will help the detox as so to will the daily salad and the main meal, the macronutrient meal, should be fulfilling and should give enough calories, so as to help maintain the body.

At the same time everyone is different and so you might want to opt for 4 meals a day or 5 meals a day or 2 meals day. But the thing is to try to avoid the foods which have been listed as not so good and to take on average one third of meals in liquid form (as in vegetable juice or smoothie) one meal as a salad and one normal main meal (but without the starchy carbs and cereals).

If you stay fairly true to this diet you wild definitely have a great detox. Taking 28 days out to avoid starchy carbs and cereals, which are prone to gut sensitivity issues, will greatly help to make an easy time for the intestines. The juices and smoothies will remove a lot of toxins, while putting in a lot of vitamins and mineral, thus helping to restore balance and rebuild the gut. Furthermore the large salad will again help with the detox, rebalance and rebuild. While the main macronutrient meal will help to maintain, strengthen and rebuild the body.

97

You might also have noticed that I haven't outlined each day and each meal and this is because it's two restrictive. Mix and match as you need to while trying to avoid the foods quoted earlier and taking one third of your food intake as vegetable liquid, one third as salad and one third as main meal.

It's a very simple yet very detoxifying meal plan. Although it's not without it challenges, as it's a low carbohydrate diet, which will make the first few days challenging. A sudden drop in carbs will make you feel weak and possibly dizzy and also maybe hungry or having lots of sugar cravings, although it will also aid for quick weight loss.

Also another challenge is the lack of beverages and snacks. We human beings are creatures of habit and apart from obvious hunger pangs; we can also suffer from withdrawal pangs. So a good idea is to have some healthy snacks handy. Nuts, raisins, prunes, currants and other such healthy snacks can be imbibed. Also certain fruits can be taken such as apples, bananas and pears. However, bananas while good for the gut, are slow to digest and can result in too much mucus if many of them are eaten. So try to keep snacking, even healthy snacks, like the fruits mentioned above to a minimum. So there's no point, for example, been on a detox and then eating 10 bananas at one sitting!

Finally stick with it for 28 days or at least until you feel you have had enough of the restriction!

If you do it right certainly a big improvement in symptoms will be noted. But also remember to keep up the maintenance. Slowly include a wide variety of foods, over the period of a few days and adjust accordingly. Don't just go back to eating the way you used to eat, as all the good work which you have achieved, over a period of weeks, can be unravelled within a few days!

Finally, it's not necessary for most people to do this 28 day program. Obviously the 28 day program will kick start your gut restoration, but it's easy to get carried away with the gimmicky idea of healing the gut within 28 days. Even if you stick with the program for 28 days, afterwards maintenance is vitally important and this is the most important part of the gut healing program. Whether or not you try out the 28 day protocol, make a point of working on detoxing, rebalancing and rebuilding and be patient enough to keep it up, over a period of months, in order to produce a long-term improvement in gut health!

Thank You

I hope you have enjoyed this book and found it interesting. These herbs, supplements and lifestyle changes are very powerful and are a simple way to support you through the recovery process. But do remember they are a support so don't simply swap allopathic medications for herbs. Pharmaceuticals, herbal formulations and lifestyle changes are simply there to assist you while you recover.

If you like this book please leave a review for it on my amazon author page!

And for more interesting and helpful information, on every suspect of physical, mental, emotional and spiritual health, please visit my website:

healbodymindandspirit.com

Thanks once again for taking the time out to read this book.

Yours in health

Dermot Farrell

About the Author

Dermot Farrell was born and raised in Ireland. He first took an interest in mental health back in the 1990's when he studied psychoanalytic studies, hypnotherapy and clinical psychoanalytical psychotherapy. While he learned a great deal about the workings of the mind, at this time, his interest in healing encouraged him to attend classes in Traditional Chinese Medicine and Acupuncture, finally culminating in a clinical diploma in 2005.

Since then he has run a TCM (Traditional Chinese Medical) clinic for a considerable period of time and also has taken to writing about a variety of topics.

Dermot has learned, from experience, the importance of balance in the three key domains of our life, which are physical, mental-emotional and spiritual well-being. His approach to healing is infinitely practical and is based upon the need to balance each of these aspects of our life, in order to regain a balanced state.

Furthermore, Dermot is interested in moving the western/eastern medical discourse forward. Believing in the virtue of both western (allopathic) and eastern (complementary) healing systems, he is continually pushing for an integrated approach to healing. As the old saying goes "doctors differ, patients die!" demonstrates the need for everyone, who is interested in health and healing, to work together towards learning more about the causes of ill-health, and the techniques of re-balancing health and reaching out in a humanistic way, so as to help patients regain their health.

As well as his interest in healing, he possesses an interest in spirituality too. In 1999 he began his meditation journey, in an Indian system of Raja Yoga, known as Sahaj Marg. With an ardent interest in spirituality as well as physical, mental and emotional healing, Dermot is presently residing in India with his wife and son.

Dermot has a website (healbodymindandspirit.com) where he writes articles about these topics.